Healthcare Security Field Manual: Patient Violence Prevention & Mitigation

HSFM 1-1.0

David Corbin

I dedicate this field manual to my wife, Shelby Ortega, whose unconditional love and support drives, nurtures, and sustains me; to my daughter, Neve, who inspires me to create a safer world for her and our future generations; and to my friend and mentor, Bonnie Michelman, whose guidance and support has been a constant source of inspiration throughout my career.

PREFACE

I wrote this field manual to provide healthcare security leaders and other healthcare leaders charged with preventing and mitigating patient violence with a resource to guide their efforts. Honestly, I felt driven to write this manual. Every time I read a news article about a healthcare worker being violently attacked, my heart sinks. It's probably because I spent over two decades of my career leading security and workplace violence programs to protect staff, patients, and visitors in both community hospitals and at a Level 1 urban trauma center. It's also because I have experienced the impacts of patient violence firsthand as a frontline responder, as a leader guiding an organization past the trauma of a recent murder/suicide on campus, and as the husband of a clinical psychologist who feared for her safety almost daily during her training. And now, my security consulting work primarily involves helping healthcare organizations to unravel the complex and evolving issues driving violence against staff. In short, I am regularly immersed in the issue of violence in healthcare in all of its forms.

I have developed a deep understanding of what works and what doesn't work when it comes to patient violence prevention and mitigation both as a practitioner and as a consultant, so I wanted to share my knowledge with healthcare leaders who can make a real impact. While writing this manual, I endeavored to back up my material with research to ensure that my own experiences, perceptions, and preconceived notions weren't the only points of reference. Through the research process, I learned a great deal more about what drives patient violence and what programs are effective. I also found that there is a startling lack of comprehensive research on patient violence prevention and mitigation, particularly regarding which strategies and tactics are effective. The relevant research that I did find, however, has been analyzed, digested, and included in this manual in the clearest terms possible.

While many healthcare organizations don't publicize it, the specter of patient violence constantly hangs heavy in the air in every patient care unit, outpatient clinic, and elsewhere across their facilities, especially for those who work in direct patient care roles. It's not that healthcare organizations aren't trying to address this violence. In fact, there are many interventions, training options, and technologies to choose from to prevent and mitigate patient violence and so many paths to take on the journey to achieve these goals. However, the sheer number of options can become overwhelming. In the process of seeking effective tactics and other interventions, many healthcare leaders miss the strategy behind implementing an effective patient violence prevention and mitigation (PVPM) program. That is why I wrote this field manual to provide a clear, multi-step process to guide the efforts of healthcare security leaders and anyone else who has joined the mission to prevent and mitigate patient violence. My hope is that the material in this manual makes a real difference in your organization. Thank you for taking on this important mission.

DISCLAIMER

Please note that every healthcare organization, its operations, challenges, and its facilities are different. While this manual provides a roadmap to build a patient violence prevention and mitigation program, each organization should assess its own situation, threats, vulnerabilities, and risks.

Implementing the PVPM program outlined in this manual does not guarantee positive outcomes. It is ultimately up to the organization to make an ongoing commitment to this program, to customize it to their needs, and to nurture and update it to address the dynamic nature of risk in the healthcare environment.

The author and Dynamic Security Strategies, LLC, disclaim any liability for personal injury, property, or any other damages of any nature whatsoever, whether special, indirect, consequential, or compensatory, directly or indirectly resulting from the publication, use of, application, or reliance on this manual. The author and Dynamic Security Strategies, LLC disclaim and make no guarantee or warranty, expressed or implied, as to the accuracy or completeness of any information published herein, and disclaim and make no warranty that the information in the document will fulfill any person's or entity's particular purposes or needs. Anyone using this document should rely on their own independent judgment or, as appropriate, seek the advice of a competent professional in determining the exercise of reasonable care in any given circumstances.

Contents

INTRODUCTION

On a near-daily basis, you can read news stories about violent assaults in healthcare facilities. These stories are often accompanied by promises from the impacted organization to "beef up security." However, these post-incident efforts are often misguided, disjointed, and, in some cases, amount to what can only be described as security theater. Rushing toward solutions in the aftermath of a serious, newsworthy incident is an understandable reaction in the wake of such trauma. But the likelihood that any of these knee-jerk reactions will result in a comprehensive and sustainable patient violence prevention program is slim to none. The threat of patient violence is not going away, but with the right prevention and mitigation efforts, this threat can be greatly reduced.

But why is this field manual focused on preventing and mitigating patient violence and not all forms of violence in healthcare? It's because patients are statistically the most frequent aggressors in healthcare, followed by visitors, coworkers, and persons with no legitimate relationship to the organization, such as those persons who are only there to commit violence (Bureau of Labor Statistics, 2013). Concentrating on the issue of patient violence instead of all forms of violence in healthcare brings the strategies and tactics that lead to the greatest reductions in harm to staff into sharp focus. The good news is that the strategies contained within this manual will also help form a solid platform upon which to build out the rest of your workplace violence program. When you get into the PVPM program portion of the manual, you'll see exactly what I mean.

This manual is primarily written with healthcare security leaders as the primary audience because these leaders are most often the ones charged with creating and driving the workplace violence prevention and mitigation program. However, many healthcare security leaders don't fully understand how to ensure that the program they are building is on solid ground or whether it's truly effective. They might be approaching the massive threat of patient violence with little to no support, few financial resources, and, at times, little buy-in from senior leadership. To be sure, patient violence and other types of violence within a healthcare organization are not issues that can be solved by one person or even one department. It takes the strength, support, engagement, and coordination of an entire organization—starting from the top—to build and sustain an impactful program. A healthcare security leader, equipped with the right support and the step-by-step strategic approach outlined in this field manual, can truly make a difference.

I decided on the field manual approach based on my experience with US Army field manuals during my time as an Army Reservist. They are no-nonsense publications that can be read and understood by anyone from a five-star general to a rank-and-file soldier. They provide valuable information on various topics, cutting to the essential information that the reader must understand in order to be effective. It is my hope that this field manual provides the same qualities and value to you. I plan to author additional field manuals in the future that address other types of violence and violence-related topics in the healthcare sector.

You may be tempted to skip directly to the part of this book that describes how to build the patient violence prevention and mitigation program, but I implore you to read the manual in its entirety to understand all of the factors that play into patient violence. After all, you can't address patient violence effectively if you don't fully understand what is causing it. Below is a quick outline of what to expect from this book as you make your way through it.

Chapter 1 describes the healthcare operational environment, starting with definitions of key concepts before moving on to the operational variables that can and will impact the effectiveness of your PVPM program strategy. Understanding these variables and what they mean for your program will help you to capitalize on organizational strengths and work with or around organizational challenges. Trust me; it's better to know what variables are playing into or against your program before you embark on your journey.

In **Chapter 2**, the foundations of patient violence in healthcare are covered. I have digested some complex information and narrowed it down to the essentials that you need to understand. This chapter and the content within will form the underpinnings of your understanding of what drives patient violence—from biological factors to socioeconomic factors and more. It will also hopefully help dispel some common misconceptions about the role of psychological factors and the propensity for patient violence. Fully understanding the issue of patient violence will ultimately empower you to lead the strategic approach to effectively preventing and mitigating it.

Chapter 3 discusses the manifestations of patient violence. The typical types of patient violence in the healthcare setting are covered along with the catalysts that can trigger violence.

After reading the first three chapters, you are ready to delve into the Patient Violence Prevention and Mitigation (PVPM) Program in **Chapter 4**. This in-depth chapter covers the four essential steps needed to build a sustainable and effective program to prevent and mitigate patient violence: Assess, Establish the Foundation, Build, and Maintain. Each step is described using the analogy of building a house to provide you with a way to visualize the program and the importance of following each step in a sequence.

Once you've read this manual, you'll have a clear understanding of how you can build a PVPM program in your own organization. And, because it is written in a field manual style, you can easily reference it as needed when you need reminders and guidance on the process. My goal here is to educate and empower you to make a difference, one step at a time.

Chapter 1.
The Healthcare Operational Environment

The operational environment in any healthcare organization is inherently complex. When you think about it, every healthcare organization is responsible for maintaining the health of its patients and navigating difficult medical, psychological, socioeconomic, biological, and other issues. There's also the omnipresence of life-and-death scenarios playing out daily. What other industry can you think of that can introduce a new human to the world on the same day that another human dies and several others are spared from death through lifesaving care? Healthcare is truly a unique industry, but it is also one filled with risk, conflict, and the ever-present risk of violence.

Oftentimes, when a leader is seeking to launch a program to prevent or mitigate patient violence, they gloss over some or all of the operational variables at play that can help or hurt their cause. Indeed, these variables can impact your organization's level of risk and vulnerability to the threat of patient violence. The key here is not just to understand these variables but to understand how you might leverage them to your advantage, overcome them if they are an obstacle, mitigate their effects, or improve them so that they better support the PVPM program. As you work through this chapter, you should take the time to write down how each of these variables applied to your organization, for better or worse (and everything in between). Then examine your notes to determine where you may need to focus your energy when building an environment supportive of your PVPM program aspirations.

Section 1. Operational Variables

Below is a list of the most common variables impacting the healthcare environment and, therefore, your efforts to stem the risk and your vulnerability to patient violence within your organization.

    A. Political: This variable includes internal and external political forces. An example of an internal political force may be a C-Suite that is eager to make the hospital safer from violence but is primarily interested in tangible security measures such as cameras, duress alarms, and metal detectors instead of other interventions that are more impactful. An example of external political force is the demonization and targeting of healthcare personnel that occurred during COVID-19 as a result of misinformation and conspiracy theories being perpetuated by some politicians.

B. **Security:** The capabilities of the security team play a significant role in influencing the degree to which patient violence prevention and mitigation (PVPM) efforts succeed. The capabilities of the team are not just limited to the number of security personnel but also refer to the training, knowledge, background, equipment, and expertise that the team brings to the table. There is no doubt that the number of security staff available to any security leader has the ability to influence the success of PVPM efforts. However, a large number of security personnel does not necessarily equate to an effective team. The overall quality of staff plays a major role in their effectiveness and drives success. A small team composed of engaged, experienced, educated, well-trained, and physically fit/able staff is much more effective than a team without some or all of these characteristics. When it comes to PVPM, the approach from security should always be "smarter, not harder."

The support for the security team, large or small, is just as critical. Support comes from internal sources, such as the C-Suite, department leadership, and individual managers and staff members, and from external sources, such as the local police. A close, collaborative working relationship with a responsive law enforcement agency can be an asset to the organization, while a contentious relationship with an agency with few resources to respond to calls for service and emergencies can add risk to the organization.

Ultimately, if PVPM efforts are to succeed, a security leader must leverage all available support resources at their disposal. Security alone cannot accomplish the PVPM mission in a vacuum. Strategies and tactics launched from an isolated, unsupported security department with a "go it alone" mentality are doomed to fail.

C. **Community:** Identifying and analyzing the community you serve is critical. You cannot succeed in PVPM without knowing your community. Every healthcare organization's community is different, but almost every community includes staff, patients, visitors, volunteers, contractors, vendors, students, interns, and more. It is essential that you understand each segment of the community and how they may (or may not) factor into your PVPM strategies and tactics.

When analyzing the impacts of PVPM strategies and tactics on the community, consider multiple perspectives: the internal perspective, including staff, volunteers, students, interns, etc.; the patient perspective; and the external perspective, including visitors, vendors, and contractors. This analysis should be used to determine the effects of PVPM efforts on the community and on patients. Each of these community categories can potentially be a source of support for PVPM efforts.

A classic example of perspective-taking relates to metal detectors at hospital entrances. Staff will likely feel safer knowing that there are metal detectors helping to keep weapons out of the hospital. However, patients may see the metal detectors as an indicator that the hospital is not safe because they perceive that people are trying to bring weapons into the facility to do harm.

D. **Economic:** This is another variable that has both an internal and external component. The finances of the healthcare organization impact its ability not only to fund security personnel and electronic security measures but may also impact its ability to fund training, provide adequate clinical staffing, and maintain facilities. A healthcare organization in financial distress will most likely turn its focus to survival and core operations, which may negatively impact the PVPM mission. External economic forces can adversely impact the organization's finances as well by impacting the ability of patients to pay for services. These forces may also lead to increases in joblessness, poverty, mental health crises, and crime in the surrounding service area of the organization, increasing the chances that these risk factors for violence are infused into the patient population.

E. **Social:** The issues within society that are impacting local, state, and national community populations are not confined to the area outside the four walls of the healthcare organization. Patients do not drop the impacts of societal issues at the door when they enter your facility. In fact, your organization may be at the heart of a particular societal issue, such as the COVID-19 pandemic, which brought both praises of healthcare heroes and suspicion among some groups and individuals who were convinced that hospitals were part of a government conspiracy to artificially inflate the impacts of the pandemic. Regardless of the societal issues at hand, their influence on your efforts to reduce and prevent violence must be examined and incorporated into any such plans.

F. **Information:** Information from internal and external sources is critical in driving decision-making, determining levels of violence risk, examining whether PVPM efforts are effective, and more. Internal sources of information include leadership and line staff, security incident reports and daily logs, clinical data like average length of stay in the emergency department, frequency of physical restraint application, patient complaints, and risk management reports. External sources of data include crime rates, trends, and risk levels sourced from law enforcement or professional crime reports, open source intelligence from news outlets and social media, and more.

G. **Infrastructure:** The infrastructure of the organization's facilities can impact PVPM measures by hindering the ability to support a safe and secure environment. Aging infrastructure, including the physical buildings, Heating, Ventilation, and Air Conditioning (HVAC), computer networks and Wi-Fi, two-way radio equipment, and patient care units with design issues can make it harder to stem the tide of violence. A persistent HVAC issue on an inpatient unit in the summer can make patient rooms too warm, leaving them feeling more agitated and unhappy. A lack of good Wi-Fi coverage in the facility can make it impossible to implement body-worn panic buttons for staff. The examples are endless in this category. If you are in an aging facility with strained financial resources, you undoubtedly have many more examples to add.

H. **Physical Environment:** The physical size and layout of the organization's campus, which includes buildings and grounds, can impact the effectiveness of PVPM efforts. A large, disconnected urban hospital campus spread across several city blocks with multiple high-rise buildings presents a greater challenge to PVPM efforts than a smaller community hospital with only three floors. The impact of the physical environment must be considered when determining—and reality-checking—PVPM strategies and tactics.

Further, the design of the physical environment plays a role in supporting violence prevention and mitigation measures. For example, a well-lit, well-maintained parking garage with good access control measures, security cameras, and call boxes are less likely to be the scene of a violent encounter than a dimly lit, crumbling facility with broken emergency exit doors and non-functioning cameras. Also, a well-designed emergency department triage room with two exit points, a duress button, and good visual sightlines to other staff is safer than a poorly designed triage room with one exit and no duress button that is located in an isolated part of the waiting area.

I. **Time:** When it comes to tactical and strategic operations, the amount of time needed versus the amount of time allotted to the security department must be considered in any planning process. You must first understand how the organization's leadership views PVPM efforts. Do they consider these efforts to be urgent? Is there time, resources, interest, and support to go about things in a logical and organized manner? Don't be surprised if urgency, lack of time, resources, and short-term interest drive your strategies and tactics. But avoid, at all costs, being pulled into the fast-moving waters of the quick-fix mentality that can grip an organization after a seriously violent incident. In any case, ongoing two-way communication between security leadership and the organization's leadership is key to understanding expectations on both sides. These expectations and the accompanying rationale behind them (yes- sometimes there is no rational explanation, but do your best) must also be communicated to the boots-on-the-ground security team if they are to successfully execute PVPM tactics.

It is critically important to understand how these variables impact your organization if your patient violence prevention and mitigation (PVPM) initiatives are to succeed. Just because these variables don't line up in your favor does not mean that your work toward a PVPM program won't succeed. It may just mean that your strategic plan may need to be formed with an acknowledgment of the realities of your organization's operations.

Chapter 2.
Foundations of Patient Violence in Healthcare

There is no single explanation for how or why patient violence occurs—there are multiple causes and risk factors. However, in order to prevent and mitigate patient violence, we must understand how and why it happens. We also must understand institutional, societal, and personal biases and perceptions about the drivers of patient violence. Oftentimes, the blame for violence is pinned on patients in certain categories, especially those with psychological diagnoses. However, research has consistently dispelled this perception. By educating yourself on the multiple factors that play into the likelihood of a patient committing an act of violence, you can help ensure that your PVPM efforts and those of other leaders are based on research and facts versus perceptions.

When it comes to the causes of patient violence, they can generally be broken down into the following categories: biological, psychological, socioeconomic, operational, and environmental factors. These categories can overlap in multiple layers both within and across categories, and together, they form the foundation of patient violence in healthcare. Each of these categories is further broken down in the following sections.

Section 1. Biological Risk Factors for Violence

Biological risk factors for violence include genetics, brain structures and connections, medical diseases, neurotransmitter issues, hormones, impacts of substances, and prescribed medications (Soreff et al., 2022, pp. 1-2). These risk factors are further broken down into a high-level overview below:

1. **Genetics:** In terms of genetics, there is one particular trait that is a greater predictor of violence than any other—the male gender. According to Soreff et al. (2022), "Whether through testosterone or societal expectations, males are dramatically over-represented as perpetrators of violence" (p. 1). Other genetic issues include, but are not limited to: chromosomal abnormality (Down syndrome) and individuals with low MAO-A expression (Soreff et al., 2022, pp. 1-2). MAO-A is "...an enzyme

that normally functions…by breaking down several key neurotransmitters: serotonin, dopamine, and norepinephrine which are important in aggression, emotion and cognition" (Garcia-Aroncena, 2015, para. 4). Serotonin plays a role in aggression control as, "excess serotonin has been linked to aggression, especially in individuals living in a stressful socioeconomic environment" (Soreff et al., 2022, p. 2).

2. **Brain Structures and Connections:** Certain issues with brain structures and connections have been linked with aggressive behavior. The prefrontal cortex serves as the executive functioning control center for the central nervous system. Executive functioning includes working memory, mental flexibility, and self-control (Harvard University, n.d., para 2). However, "Reduced activity of the prefrontal cortex…is associated with violent aggression" (Soreff et al., 2022, p. 2). Another example of an issue with the prefrontal cortex and executive functioning is Alzheimer's disease, which impacts this area of the brain and "can remove the inhibitions normally applied and result in unchecked aggressive activity" (Soreff et al., 2022, p. 2). According to the Alzheimer's Association, "Aggression can be caused by many factors, including physical discomfort, environmental factors, and poor communication" (Alzheimer's Association, n.d., para. 2).

3. **Medical Diseases:** Not all medical diseases result in aggression, but certain diseases can increase the likelihood of violence. There is one particular medical condition that is most important in causing aggression—pain. When it comes to pain, "Regardless of the physical origin of the pain, the person often strikes out in response to the unbearable discomfort" (Soreff et al., 2022, p. 2). Other examples of medical diseases and conditions that can result in aggression include epilepsy and patients in respiratory distress. Epileptic patients whose disease originates in the temporal or frontal lobes have exhibited violence (Soreff et al., 2022, p. 2). Patients who are in breathing distress from asthma or chronic obstructive pulmonary disease (COPD) have been known to become aggressive (Soreff et al., 2022, p. 2).

4. **Neurotransmitter Issues:** According to Soreff et al. (2022), "Several neurotransmitters have been linked to aggressive behavior, usually when they are excessive or deficient. Serotonin in both excess and deficiency has been correlated with aggression…Low serotonin has been correlated with depression, violence, and

suicide" (p. 2). However, according to Krakowski (2003), "There is no one-to-one relationship between serotonin and aggression, but rather a complex interplay among various factors. Aggressive behavior cannot be easily dissociated from impulse control, affect regulation, and social functioning" (p. 302). Aggression can also be triggered by excess dopamine. People with schizophrenia and those with Parkinson's often have high levels of dopamine, with the latter experiencing high dopamine levels from medication to compensate for loss of dopamine cells (Soreff et al., 2022; Zahoor & Haq, 2018).

5. **Hormones:** As stated earlier, testosterone can drive aggressive behavior in males. However, women receiving testosterone have also been shown to become aggressive (Soreff et al., 2022, p. 2).

6. **Substances:** Several substances are known to create a greater potential for aggressive behavior and violence. In particular, alcohol, hallucinogens, PCP, and anabolic steroids are among those that have the higher potential to create violence. Alcohol reduces inhibition to controlling emotions, while hallucinogens can create frightening experiences for the users that cause them to lash out. PCP makes users feel that they have superhuman abilities and makes them impervious to pain, and may cause violent behavior. Anabolic steroids can lead to aggressive rage. Further, withdrawal from any of these and other addictive substances can make the user resort to violence in order to obtain more of the substance (Soreff et al., 2022, p. 2).

7. **Prescription Medication:** Some prescription medications can trigger aggression as a side effect. One example is antidepressants, which can lead to suicidal and homicidal behavior, especially in children. Another example is the dopamine-increasing drugs used to treat Parkinson's, mentioned earlier in this section (Soreff et al., 2022, p. 2). A 2010 study found that varenicline, otherwise known as Chantix- a drug used for smoking cessation- was linked to acts of violence towards others more strongly than thirty other prescription drugs in the study (Moore & Furberg, 2010, p. 4).

In summary, there are several risk factors related to biological conditions, some of which may not be apparent to non-medical healthcare professionals. However, these risk factors may be revealed by clinical staff during or after a violent incident or revealed within data collected after violent incidents using incident reports and other sources. The degree to which your organization is exposed to these risk factors may vary based on a variety of variables, including the patient population served and the types of services and specialties offered by your organization.

Section 2. Psychological Risk Factors for Violence

There are certain psychological diagnoses that have violent behavior indicated as part of their features. Examples include, but are not limited to, bipolar disorder, schizophrenia, dementia, post-traumatic stress disorder (PTSD), and acute stress disorder (Soreff et al., 2022, pp. 2-3). In children and adolescents, intellectual deficiencies, some personality disorders, and intermittent explosive disorder are linked to violence.

However, there is often stigma unfairly attached to patients with psychological diagnoses where they are presumed to be dangerous and more likely to become violent. According to the National Alliance on Mental Illness (NAMI) (n.d), "Stigma is when someone, or even you yourself, views a person in a negative way just because they have a mental health condition. Some people describe stigma as a feeling of shame or judgment [sic] from someone else" (para. 1). In healthcare, patients with psychological diagnoses or those in crisis exhibiting symptoms consistent with psychological diagnoses are sometimes referred to by clinicians and/or security staff as "psych" or "psych patients" — a dehumanizing term that typically comes with the attached violence risk stigma. The impact of this stigma, according to Knaak et al. (2017), is that "People with lived experience of a mental illness commonly report feeling devalued, dismissed, and dehumanized by many of the health professionals with whom they come into contact" (p. 111).

Studies examining the risk of violence in people with psychiatric diagnoses have found that "the relationship between mental illness and violence has been shown to be more complex than initially suspected" (Varshney et al., 2016, p. 223). In fact, when researchers reanalyzed data from the National Epidemiologic Survey on Alcohol and Related Conditions (NESARC), they found the following:

> "...mental illness and violence are related primarily through the accumulation of risk factors of various kinds, for example, historical (past violence, juvenile detention, physical abuse, parental arrest record), clinical (substance abuse,

perceived threats), dispositional (age, sex, etc.) and contextual (recent divorce, unemployment, victimization) among the mentally ill. In fact, for those with mental illness without substance use, the relationship with violence was modest at best" (Varshney et al., 2016, pp. 223-224).

It is important to note that, outside of formal psychological diagnoses, "...when people are afraid, overwhelmed, feel threatened, or feel out of control, perplexed, disorientated, or frustrated, they often respond aggressively" (Soreff et al., 2022, p. 3). These emotions and experiences are all endemic to the healthcare environment regardless of location, patient population, resources, and efforts by the organization to prevent or mitigate situations that may trigger them. For example, many patients arriving at an emergency department are afraid and overwhelmed by their symptoms and what they could mean for their health and/or their lives. Someone who wakes up from anesthesia in the post-anesthesia care unit (PACU) may be disoriented and may not know why people are standing around them in an unfamiliar environment. A patient in a doctor's office waiting room whose appointment is running twenty minutes late could get frustrated, especially if they have somewhere else to go. Just think about how often this happens in any healthcare setting every day. Not every person will react the same to these situations, but depending on a variety of factors, some will resort to violence. Below are some examples of possible psychological causes of violence:

1. **Bipolar Affective Disorder:** Bipolar affective disorder patients who are in the manic phase can exhibit aggression and agitation. This is because the manic phase includes "Grandiose delusions [that] often not only dramatically inflate their self-view but also make them demanding of others and combative to those not acknowledging their perceived greatness" (Soreff et al., 2022, p. 2).

2. **Schizophrenia:** According to Soreff et al. (2022), "Patients with schizophrenia can be aggressive when responding to command hallucinations ordering them to harm others" (pp. 2-3). Command hallucinations are described as "...auditory hallucinations that instruct a patient to act in specific ways; these commands can range in seriousness from innocuous to life-threatening" (Hersh & Borum, 1998, p. 353). However, not all patients with schizophrenia experiencing command hallucinations will act on them. A study by Scott et al. found that "Between 30% to 65% of individuals with

command hallucinations to harm others...comply with those hallucinations" (Scott & Resnick, 2017, pp. 623-632).

3. **Dementia:** As mentioned in the Biological Factors section of this manual, patients experiencing issues with their prefrontal cortex that impacts executive functioning can become aggressive and violent. Dementia and Alzheimer's, which is a form of dementia, "...not only have memory deficiencies but also lose their executive functions" (Soreff et al., 2022, p. 3). Executive functioning loss also means loss of inhibition, including inhibition of impulsive behavior, such as lashing out violently. Violence related to executive functioning loss can "...account for some of the violence seen in long-term care facilities and in places where patients with traumatic brain injuries are treated" (Soreff et al., 2022, p. 3).

4. **Post-Traumatic Stress Disorder (PTSD):** PTSD can happen to anyone experiencing trauma. In fact, for adults, the National Center for PTSD at the US Department of Veterans Affairs (2018) indicates that "About 6 out of every 100 people (or 6% of the population) will have PTSD at some point in their lives" (para. 3). For children and teens experiencing trauma, "...3% to 15% of girls and 1% to 6% of boys develop PTSD" (US Dept. of Veterans Affairs, 2018, para. 2). Further, according to Soreff et al. (2022), "Patients with PTSD struggle with a host of symptoms that can promote potential aggression. These symptoms include hypervigilance, flashbacks, and nightmares, and can lead to aggression" (p. 3).

Sadly, Veterans who have served our country in combat are often unfairly stigmatized as being more likely to have PTSD and, therefore, considered more likely to be violent. However, "the majority of Veterans and non-Veterans with PTSD have never engaged in violence" (Norman et al., 2014, para. 1). Also, the association between PTSD and violence is decreased "When other factors like alcohol and drug misuse, additional psychiatric disorders, or younger age are considered..." (Norman et al., 2014, para. 1).

5. **Childhood Diagnoses:** Regarding childhood psychological diagnoses, there are several that can result in aggressive behavior, including, but not limited to: "...conduct disorder and attention-deficit/hyperactivity disorder (ADHD), [and] disorders along the autism spectrum, because of communication difficulties, impulsiveness, low

tolerance, and frustration" (Soreff et al., 2022, p. 3). Persons with Autism Spectrum Disorder (ASD) are sometimes unfairly stigmatized as being more likely to act out violently, including in clinical settings.

However, according to a study published in the Harvard Review of Psychiatry examining the possible connection between ASD and violence:

> "Findings from descriptive case reports, prevalence studies, and previous reviews suggest that, while no conclusive evidence indicates that individuals with ASD are more violent than those without ASD, specific generative and associational risk factors may increase violence risk among individuals with ASD" (Im, 2016, p. 32).

According to the author, generative risk factors include "comorbid psychopathology, social-cognition deficits, emotion-regulation problems" (Im, 2016, p. 29), while associational risk factors include "younger age, Asperger's syndrome diagnosis, repetitive behavior" (Im, 2016, p. 14).

6. **Intellectual Deficiencies and Personality Disorders:** Persons who have intellectual deficiencies, such as Down's Syndrome, fetal alcohol syndrome, or other such deficiencies, "when confronting difficult tasks and situations, may resort to violence as a coping mechanism" (Soreff et al., 2022, p. 3). Further, individuals with antisocial personality disorders "lack an empathic view and have an egocentric center of gravity, which can promote aggression" (Soreff et al., 2022, p. 3).

   Someone with a borderline personality disorder "who is overwhelmed and has boundary issues can become aggressive" (Soreff et al., 2022, p. 3). However, these episodes of aggression are "...expressed particularly towards intimate partners and known persons, usually in the homes of perpetrators" (Sarkar, 2019, p. 579).

   Further, intermittent explosive disorder (IED) "...is marked by frequent and distinct episodes in which an individual fails to resist aggressive impulses or reactions grossly out of proportion to any provocation" ("Intermittent Explosive Disorder," 2022).

Again, it is important to remember that persons with psychological diagnoses are not automatically predisposed to violence. There are a number of complex factors that play into the risk of violence for anyone, including persons with psychological diagnoses. The healthcare environment can trigger emotions in any patient that can lead them to react violently. However, stigmatizing persons with mental health issues does more harm than good for the patient and the level and quality of care they receive. It can also result in the PVPM program elements being overly focused on the wrong patient population. To learn more about stigma related to mental health, visit NAMI.org and visit the StigmaFree Me page, where you can also take a stigma quiz and take a pledge to live stigma-free.

Section 3. Socioeconomic Risk Factors for Violence

A patient's socioeconomic situation is "...the position of an individual or group on the socioeconomic scale, which is determined by a combination of social and economic factors such as income, amount and kind of education, type and prestige of occupation, place of residence, and—in some societies or parts of society—ethnic origin or religious background" ("Socioeconomic Status," 2022). Healthcare organizations serve patients from a wide range of socioeconomic backgrounds. Some socioeconomic factors have been linked to the likelihood of violence. A recent study found that "...nine factors correctly classified 80% of violent patients at the time of admission..." (Pitts & Schaller, 2022, p. 1). Only three of the nine factors were related to socioeconomic status, specifically, "...no history of employment, and homelessness..." (Pitts & Schaller, 2022, p. 1). The other factors identified in the study included "...diagnosis of psychosis or bipolar disorder, history of psychiatric disorder, male gender, age younger than 35 years, below-average intelligence... and agitated behavior" (Pitts & Schaller, 2022, p. 1).

However, a patient's socioeconomic challenges, while a potential risk factor, should not be used as a primary basis for evaluating their potential for violence. Sadly, patients with lower socioeconomic status are already up against difficult challenges that are compounded by the substandard level of care they receive from healthcare organizations. A 2021 study by 3M indicated that "...an individual's socioeconomic status (SES) impacts the health care services they receive, health outcomes, patient satisfaction and physician perception of the care and treatment needed" (Averell & Mills, 2021 p. 2).

It is important that socioeconomic factors do not negatively impact the ability of patients to access quality care within a healthcare organization. Further, the violence risk factors associated with socioeconomic status should not be used against these patients when seeking care.

Section 4. Operational Risk Factors for Violence

The operations of a healthcare institution have the potential to impact the healthcare environment and, therefore, the likelihood of patient violence. A well-run healthcare facility with ample human and financial resources is more likely to have shorter wait times for patients, better staff-to-patient ratios, and the ability to attract and retain top talent. A facility without these resources may have longer wait times, overburdened clinical staff, and high turnover rates, resulting in a lower quality of care, and an elevated potential for conflict.

However, this does not mean that only facilities with ample resources can effectively prevent and mitigate patient violence. But, it might mean that facilities with fewer resources must leverage different strategies and tactics that make the best use of limited resources. Understanding your organization's operations and associated advantages or limitations is key to crafting effective PVPM strategies.

Operational factors for consideration and analysis when planning PVPM strategies and tactics include, but are not limited to, the following:

1. Staff turnover, clinical and support role vacancies, recruiting challenges.

2. Staff-to-patient ratios—both normal and current.

3. C-Suite turnover, vacancies, and impacts of interim leadership.

4. Key on-site leadership availability after normal operating hours.

5. Availability of psychological or psychiatric clinical services and support.

6. Mergers in progress with other healthcare organizations or facilities.

As you may have surmised from the items listed above, some of these operational risk factors are temporary, while others are more permanent or ingrained into the organization. For example, healthcare organizations have long strived to fill vacancies with qualified staff, but the after-effects of COVID-19 have exacerbated this situation, leading to serious staff shortages, overreliance on traveling healthcare staff, and dangerous staff-to-patient ratios. Regardless of the nature of these operational risk factors, they should be examined for their potential impacts on your PVPM program implementation and sustainability.

Section 5. Environmental Risk Factors for Violence

Operational issues can ultimately positively or negatively impact the healthcare environment. In fact, "Several studies have found a direct correlation with multiple aspects regarding the hospital setting and violent behavior" (Pitts & Schaller, 2022, p. 1). Environmental factors that have greater contributions to violence include "Long waiting times, lack of security, lack of adequate staff, and patient areas being open to the public...respectively" (Pitts & Schaller, 2022, p. 1). In the emergency department, there are additional environmental factors that contribute to the likelihood of violence, including "...increased number of patients and visitors using alcohol and drugs, psychiatric disorders, dementia, the presence of weapons, stressful environment, overcrowding, prolonged waiting times, and flow of violence from the community into the ED" (Pitts & Schaller, 2022, p.1).

Although some factors can be controlled by initial design or renovation of the built environment, added resources, and/or operational improvements, some factors leading to violence may be inherent to some healthcare environments, such as extended wait times and staffing shortages.

There are also external environmental factors that can impact the likelihood of patient violence. Most notably, a high violent crime rate in the service area surrounding the campus can result in violence spilling from the streets onto the campus and into facilities. External crime is typically beyond the control of the organization, but some hospitals have extended their reach into the community to stop the cycle of violence through innovative violence intervention initiatives. It is important to understand external, violent crime risks and any part that your hospital may play in stemming community violence as part of your PVPM program planning. Crime risk reports available from companies such as CAP Index® and SecurityGauge® are helpful in determining not only current violent crime risks but also future violent crime risks. Analysis of the causal factors of violence within and outside of your organization using available data is key to understanding which environmental factors may be contributing to the risk of violence.

Now that you have read this chapter, I urge you to re-read it and think about whether any of the information within changes your perceptions about the causes of patient violence. If it does, think about how you might approach the issue of patient violence differently with your updated perceptions and perspectives. Further, this new information might change your thinking about where patient violence is most likely to occur within your organization based on factors such as clinical specialties, specialized care units, and the types of patient populations served within your facilities.

Chapter 3.
Manifestations of Patient Violence

Patient violence can take many forms, but the primary forms are verbal and physical violence and threats. These primary forms of violence can vary in intensity. Physical violence can range from an inappropriate brush against a clinician's body part to strangulation. Verbal violence can range from inappropriate sexual language to threats of imminent violence. Threats can be veiled or overtly frightening and imminently dangerous. Violence in all of its forms is unacceptable in the healthcare environment, so efforts to prevent and mitigate it should include the full spectrum of violent behaviors.

It's important to note that the recipient of patient violence is often not the only victim involved. Staff who witness patient violence can experience trauma just from watching it unfold, feeling helpless to intervene, or just from hearing another staff member recount their experience with a violent patient. In fact, an entire healthcare organization can suffer collective trauma if there is a violent incident that results in serious injury or death.

Section 1. Primary Types of Patient Violence

1. **Verbal Violence:** Verbal violence involves threatening or abusive language towards staff and others, such as threats of harm to self or others, and racist, sexist, sexual, or otherwise demeaning and inappropriate language. This language is typically intended to place the person in imminent fear for their physical safety, intimidate or harass them.

2. **Physical Violence:** Physical violence includes both assault and battery.

    a. Assault is placing someone in imminent fear of battery. This is often accomplished by actions such as assuming a fighting stance, pointing a finger in someone's face, or attempting to grab or strike someone with a fist or foot.

    b. Battery is actually making physical contact with someone without their consent in a way that is likely to cause bodily harm and may include punching, pinching, biting, kicking, pushing, and other actions.

        i. Sexual battery is generally defined as touching the intimate part of another person (buttocks, breasts, genitals), whether clothed or unclothed, against their will for the purpose of sexual arousal, sexual gratification, or sexual abuse.

3. **Threats:** While threats can take the form of verbal or physical violence, they can also take the form of written communication through email, text, mail, and other formats. These threats may be communicated when the patient is in the care environment or after they have left. A threat can generally be defined as a statement or action that places another person in fear for their safety from physical harm.

Section 2. Additional Types of Patient Violence

1. **Murder:** While murders are thankfully rare in the healthcare environment, they are still a type of violence that must be considered in planning your PVPM program. Murder is defined by the FBI Uniform Crime Reporting (UCR) Program as "...the willful (nonnegligent) killing of one human being by another" ("Murder," 2019, para. 1). Statistics on healthcare workers murdered at the hands of patients are hard to come by, but a 2019 murder of a nurse in Baton Rouge, Louisiana, highlighted the risk. The nurse initially survived a violent attack by a patient as she tried to save the life of a co-worker who was initially the target of the patient. She later died in the same hospital from a blood clot that was determined to be a direct result of the attack (Brusie, 2022).

2. **Rape:** Rape is defined by the FBI Uniform Crime Reporting (UCR) Program as "...penetration, no matter how slight, of the vagina or anus with any body part or object, or oral penetration by a sex organ of another person, without the consent of the victim" ("Rape," 2019). While instances of rape are rare in the healthcare environment, there have been reported instances of rape or attempted rape against caregivers in the patient's room, even with another staff present, during the process of an assault and battery incident.

3. **Stalking:** Some patients may engage in stalking behaviors towards their caregiver that may begin while receiving care and continue after they have been discharged from care. Stalking is generally defined as:

> "...a course of conduct directed at a specific person that would cause a reasonable person to feel fear. Unlike other crimes that involve a single incident, stalking is a pattern of behavior...made up of individual acts that could, by themselves, seem harmless or noncriminal, but when taken in the context of a stalking situation, could constitute criminal acts" ("Stalking," 2021).

There are laws on the books in every state in the US against stalking that include the specific elements of the crime.

While patient violence sometimes rises to the level of criminality, most incidents do not result in prosecution. There are a variety of reasons that patients are not charged with crimes, including a lack of interest by the victim in pursuing criminal charges, medical or psychological impairment of the patient, reluctance or refusal by law enforcement to arrest and/or charge the patient, or lack of support by the hospital's leadership for prosecuting patients. Sometimes, there's even a misperception that the healthcare organization as an entity must press charges against a patient. However, the victim of the violence is the only one that can initiate the process of prosecuting a patient.

Ultimately, the complex factors leading to an act of patient violence, the severity of the incident, the patient's condition, and, very importantly, the victim's desire and willingness to pursue criminal charges must be considered when deciding whether or not to prosecute a patient. What's critically important is that the healthcare organization supports the victim in whatever choice they make.

Section 3. Catalysts of Patient Violence

There are situational factors and certain types of clinical events that are more likely to trigger patient violence. A 2014 study of patient violence against healthcare staff revealed that the patient's behavior accounted for 40% of violence against staff with two dominant catalysts- cognitive impairment and demanding to leave (Arnetz et al., 2015). Cognitive impairment is generally defined as "problems people have with cognitive functions such as thinking, reasoning, memory, or attention" (Roy, 2013, p. 449).

The study also found that patient care that involved physically touching the patient was also a catalyst for violence, specifically situations involving needles, procedures that caused pain or discomfort, and/or where there was a need to transfer the patient from one location to another, such as from a wheelchair to a bed (Arnetz et al., 2015).

The final category the study identified was transitions, specifically "Restraints, Transitions, Intervening and Redirecting" (Arnetz et al., 2015, p. 8). The inclusion of restraints in this list is no surprise given that these are very physical events that are precipitated by the patient attempting to harm themselves or others. Transitions not only involved the patient moving from one physical place to another or being admitted but also transitioning out of anesthesia. Intervening involved staff, usually from security, attempting to stop a patient from acting out or hurting themselves or others. Redirecting involves staff trying to help a patient back into their room or into their bed (Arnetz et al., 2015).

It's no surprise that physically touching a patient, restricting their actual or perceived freedom, and causing them pain or discomfort can result in violence from them. It's quite likely that you have personal experiences that back up these findings. Ensuring that staff interacting with patients in these scenarios understand the elevated risk of violence is vitally important.

Chapter 4.

The Patient Violence Prevention & Mitigation Program

Section 1. Overview

In order to build a successful PVPM program, you must take a phased approach that leverages all of your available resources within the organization. As stated earlier in this manual, security alone cannot implement an effective, sustainable program. This is a complex, multifaceted issue that requires the expertise and engagement of a multidisciplinary team within the organization. However, as a healthcare security leader, you will often be placed in a position where you are charged with establishing an effective PVPM program.

Most healthcare organizations already have elements of a PVPM program in place. In many cases, these elements were added piecemeal to address patient violence or other security issues as they rose to the top of the organization's priorities in response to a seriously violent incident and/or due to the initiative of an individual or group. However, the issue with a piecemeal approach is that there are often disjointed elements of a workplace violence program that don't quite fit together right, lack a foundation, or simply don't add up to a coherent PVPM program that is truly effective. If a program is to succeed at addressing the complex issue of patient violence, it must be built on a solid foundation and follow the strategy outlined within this chapter.

Before launching a program, you must define what success looks like and how you'll determine whether your program is successful (you'll need data). Short and long-term strategic planning is key here, as you're not going to be able to do everything at once. In fact, trying to launch a program too quickly can backfire since it will likely end up looking and feeling like it was slapped together haphazardly. While there may be pressure to move forward quickly, an effective program must be carefully built over a period of time with the right support and a focused, strategic, long-range view of the future state of safety and security that you are working to create.

Section 2. The PVPM Program

The PVPM program is based on a four-step process: Assess, Establish the Foundation, Build, and Maintain. This process is meant to ensure that the program is based on data and research, has a solid footing and support, includes the elements necessary to stem the tide of patient violence, and is sustainable.

For organizations that already have established elements of a PVPM program, this process does not necessarily mean that the program must be torn down and rebuilt. Instead, the organization should use the process to assess their program to determine what elements are missing or were skipped in the process of developing it. This assessment may result in the need to: make some tweaks to the program to shore up its foundation, perform a gut renovation, or tear it down and start over. In other cases, it may mean that the program needs to be defragmented, meaning that the pieces of the program need to be reorganized to fit into the program, which will create a clear picture of what pieces of the program are still missing.

The steps in the PVPM program process are explained in more detail below. In order to help you visualize and understand the process, we'll use the analogy of building a house to explain each step. Figure 1 lays out the steps and the tasks within each step that make up the PVPM program.

1. **Assess:** The assessment step is like surveying the land before the house is built. You can't build a house on land that won't support it, and you can't begin to build a PVPM program without data and information to support it. An assessment to support a PVPM program should leverage available relevant data related to patient violence, institutional information, and research.

2. **Establish the Foundation:** Once your assessment is complete and you are clear on why and how you need to build your program to ensure it is on stable ground, you will need to establish the program's foundation. Like the ground it's built on, a solid foundation is necessary to build a stable, firmly-rooted house. This program must also have a solid base of support, multidisciplinary participation, and the organizational drive to sustain it.

3. **Build:** After the foundation is established, it's time to build the core of the house, er, program. In the build step, the operational, strategic, and tactical elements that make

Maintain

Repeat PVPM program steps annually

Conduct ongoing unit-level assessments

Leverage micro-training

Build

Take action on your assessment

Designate a PVPM program leader

Establish/evaluate your training program

Create Threat Assessment/Management Team

Establish patient behavioral emergency response and management framework

Investigate incidents and support victims

Mitigate forensic patient risk

Get a seat at the new construction/renovation planning table

Create a data visualization dashboard

Establish the Foundation

Obtain C-Suite support and engagement

Befriend the communications team

Establish a workplace violence committee

Develop policies and procedures

Assess   Understand the issues of patient violence

Gather and analyze data

Conduct a patient violence risk assessment, develop recommendations

Fig. 1 - Patient Violence Prevention and Mitigation (PVPM) Outline

the program function are added in a phased, logical way. The build step creates the core of your program, including the day-to-day operations, and establishes a *bias for action with a basis in data* approach to addressing patient violence.

4. **Maintain:** Think of the maintain step like adding a roof to the house to protect what you have built from the elements and then continuously checking the house from the foundation up for any issues and addressing them. The same idea applies to your PVPM program. Once you have worked so diligently to build it, you don't want to simply "set it and forget it," as the program will need regular assessment and maintenance to stay both effective and current.

Section 3. PVPM Program Step 1: Assess

Prior to building your PVPM program, you will need to assess the issue of patient violence within your organization. There are several ways you can do this, but this process must be done using a multidisciplinary approach. You won't have all of the information that you need to perform an effective assessment at your fingertips. Further, you will very likely need to engage the assistance of other professionals in your organization to help you tabulate and analyze the information you have gathered. With that being said, here are the elements of the assessment step:

1. Understand the Issue of Patient Violence: Review chapters 1-3 to help you understand the healthcare operational environment, the foundations of patient violence in healthcare, and the manifestations and catalysts of patient violence. Then seek to understand how these factors apply to your organization, your department, resources, and other factors related to patient violence. You cannot begin to assess or address patient violence before you understand it.

2. Gather Data: Obtain data from a variety of sources going back about three years to ensure that your lens on patient violence incidents and factors isn't too narrow. Data sources may include, but are not limited to: security incident reports, risk management reports, occupational health injury reports, patient complaints, restraint, and seclusion data, staff surveys, staff exit interviews, and more. Gaps or shortcomings in data collection are an opportunity to make improvements for the future. As the saying goes, "garbage in, garbage out." If you collect good data consistently, it will yield better insights.

3. Analyze Data: Once you have gathered your data, you'll want to analyze it. You're analyzing the data to gather the following key insights:

   a. The number of violent incidents by patients by type (verbal, physical) and trends.

   b. The scope of violence- where and when (day/time/shift) it is happening, frequency of occurrence, who it's happening to, and associated trends.

   c. Causal factors of violence- if it can be determined by data, determine the reported causes of violence or the circumstances of the violent incident. What was happening before the violent incident erupted?

   d. The severity of violence- injuries inflicted upon staff by patients and how many lost workdays are associated with these injuries. Note that it is much more difficult to determine the psychological impacts on staff who are victims of violence or have witnessed violence from data as these issues most often go unreported. However, it is important to understand that psychological trauma is happening and is a factor in evaluating the impacts of patient violence. Keep in mind that violent incidents against staff are underreported by staff, so the data you have likely does not reflect the true prevalence of patient violence.

4. Conduct a Patient Violence Risk Assessment: Review the physical and procedural security related to patient violence prevention and mitigation across patient care areas within the organization using the data you analyzed to focus your assessment priorities. Tour and assess the areas where violence is most prevalent in more depth, but don't neglect to visit and assess other areas where patient violence is possible, such as outpatient clinics, the cashier's office, and the outpatient pharmacy. You're looking for things like unit-level access control, staff access to duress alarms, de-escalation training saturation among staff, and patient room design elements that support staff safety. As part of your assessment, speak with leadership and staff across the organization to understand what their experiences are regarding patient violence. The information you gather from interviews will help bring the data you analyzed to life by adding context.

For guidance on how to conduct a risk assessment, reference the 2015 ANSI/ASIS/RIMS Risk Assessment Standard, available at www.asisonline.org in the Standards

& Guidelines section of the website. At the time of this publication, the standard is being offered at no cost in response to the COVID-19 pandemic.

5. Create Recommendations to Mitigate Identified Issues: Once you have completed all of the elements of the "assess" step, it is time to digest all of the information you have gathered and determine the next steps. Your assessment and analysis of the data should be used to develop a list of prioritized recommendations to mitigate the vulnerabilities, risks, and threats you identified. The recommendations should be based, in part, on sound or best practices, empirically validated effective interventions, regulatory compliance, local, state, and federal laws, and accreditation standards. These recommendations, combined with the next steps within the PVPM program, will drive your organization's efforts going forward to address patient violence.

Section 4. PVPM Program Step 2: Establish the Foundation

Now it's time to establish a sound foundation for your PVPM program. This is by far the most important and challenging part of the program, not because it requires a heavy monetary investment but because it requires a heavy organizational commitment. Here are the key elements that should be in place to establish a foundation:

1. **C-Suite Support and Engagement:** The single most important element of your program's foundation is obtaining the full, visible, and unwavering support of the PVPM program from your organization's senior leadership team. From the President & Chief Executive Officer to the Chief Nursing Officer and Chief Financial Officer, there must be 100% buy-in for the program. This support can't only be confined to the aftermath of a seriously violent incident or other efforts to "put out a fire" related to violence. It must be consistent, and it must be visible to the organization through regular organization-wide and targeted communications from the C-Suite to demonstrate the importance of PVPM. However, in order to get the support of the C-Suite, you first need to educate them on the risk and impacts of patient violence in your organization. This is where all of your efforts in the "assess" step come into play. Use the information you gathered and analyzed, along with your recommendations from the patient violence risk assessment, to make a case for making PVPM a priority.

2. **Find a Champion:** Within the C-Suite, it is important to find someone who is willing to champion the PVPM efforts through their direct support, guidance, and advice. Ideally, this person should be in a clinical or clinical-adjacent leadership role. This person will be absolutely key in shepherding the program forward, overcoming or removing barriers, and keeping the rest of the C-Suite engaged and informed.

3. **Befriend the Communications Team:** The communications team, or public relations/ public affairs team as it is called in some organizations, is crucial to engage in your efforts to build a successful PVPM program. Not only can they help communicate the great PVPM work that is happening within the organization to staff and leadership, but they can also help you leverage their expertise in developing educational videos, messaging campaigns, and more. They are an invaluable resource to your efforts, and their support is paramount.

4. **Establish a Workplace Violence Committee:** The Workplace Violence Committee should be a multidisciplinary group of leaders with select staff participants from across disciplines. The mission of this committee should be to use their collective expertise to drive the PVPM program and other workplace violence prevention and mitigation efforts forward. The committee should also regularly educate itself on internal and external trends related to workplace violence through formal training and research. An appropriate committee charter and governance structure should also be established with regular reporting to the C-Suite and the Board.

5. **Develop Policies & Procedures:** One of the first charges of the Workplace Violence Committee should be to review existing policies and procedures related to patient violence and other forms of violence within the organization. A gap analysis should be conducted to determine if there are any additional policies or procedures that are needed. Redundant policies should also be identified and addressed. Current policies in place should be reviewed to determine if they are current, effective, based on sound or best practices and empirically validated effective interventions, and compliant with regulations, local, state, and federal laws, and accreditation standards. Once the review process has been completed, the committee should work on developing or revising policies and procedures as needed. All new or revised policies and procedures should be communicated to leadership, then to staff within the organization.

Section 5. PVPM Program Step 3: Build

Now that your foundation has been established, you can move on to the "build" step of the program. It can be tempting to skip right to the "build" step instead of assessing and/or establishing a foundation since building the program can yield more tangible, tactical-level results. But without taking the previous two steps, your PVPM program will be on shaky footing at best and will not be nearly as effective or sustainable as it could be. If you're being pressured by leadership to build first and then add a foundation and assess, it's important that you explain why this is a bad idea and a bandage approach to a systemic issue. Below you will find the core elements you should consider for the "build" step. Note that these are core elements that will give you the most return on your efforts, and many of these elements will serve to help prevent or mitigate not only patient violence but other types of violence as well.

You'll notice that security technology is not included in this section. There are two reasons for this: 1) The determination of what security technology is needed in various areas will be based primarily on that area's risk, existing technology, and environmental factors; 2) Currently, there is little to no research supporting the idea that security technology such as duress alarms, security cameras, body-worn cameras, and other similar technology prevent or mitigate violence (Barak et al., 2016; Braga et al., 2018; Perkins et al., 2017; Piza et al., 2019). This is not to say that security technology doesn't play a role in the overall protection of the healthcare environment. This technology is an important part of any layered approach to security. However, an overreliance on technology as a means to prevent patient violence and other types of violence is very unlikely to yield positive results.

The core elements of the "build" step are as follows:

1. **Take action on your assessment:** With your foundation established, you should move forward with the prioritized recommendations you developed as a result of your patient violence risk assessment using a phased approach. This is a critical element of the "build" step and is also an opportunity for you and the team that conducted the assessment to build credibility. If you simply conduct an assessment and then throw it on a shelf to be dusted off later when something bad happens, all of

your work is in vain. Here are some considerations for how to take action to address the findings of your assessment:

a. Ensure that your recommendations are prioritized by the level of risk they present to people, assets, and/or the organization as a whole and not by internal politics or the latest fire that needs to be extinguished.

b. Address the recommendations that you identified as top priorities first, focusing on those that yield "the most bang for the buck." You will find that the recommendations that fit this category are often inexpensive or cost nothing to implement. However, they very often require a great deal of coordination, buy-in, and multidisciplinary engagement. But if you established a firm foundation for your program, these hurdles should be easier to overcome.

c. Don't neglect the quick wins that you may be able to realize by tackling lower-priority items that are simple and quick to implement. For example, adding "no weapons allowed" signs to all entry points into your facilities can demonstrate your commitment to a safe workplace. Just be sure that you have a policy in place regarding weapons and that this policy has been communicated across the organization. Otherwise, these signs are just security theater.

d. Request capital investments using a phased approach. If your recommendations require capital investments, such as a mass communications system, access control systems, duress alarms, and more, these can be overwhelming requests for any organization. By offering a phased approach based on priority levels, you can offer a predictable investment request each fiscal year for the improvements that are based on a multi-year improvement plan.

e. Report PVPM improvements to the appropriate committees and leadership. Ensure that the environment of care committee, workplace violence committee, and key leadership are regularly informed of improvements that impact PVPM and support staff and patient safety.

f. Celebrate wins. When you implement a new workplace violence policy, implement access control for your inpatient units, roll out de-escalation training across the organization, or make other improvements that positively impact PVPM, be sure to celebrate these wins. One of the best ways to do this is to engage your communications team to highlight what you've done. Don't forget to push these wins out to the public as well, where appropriate.

2. **Designate a PVPM Program Leader:** It is critically important that an appropriate leader within the organization is identified and empowered to lead both the PVPM program and other workplace violence prevention and mitigation efforts. Oftentimes, the program leader is the Director of Security. However, some organizations are creating distinct and focused roles for these leaders, with the title of "Director of Workplace Violence Prevention" or similar.

   Further, the Joint Commission, in their updated workplace violence standards, under Leadership Standard LD.03.01.01-EP 9, requires that "The hospital has a workplace violence prevention program led by a designated individual…" ("Violence Prevention Standards," 2021, p. 4). The designated individual may be the security director or someone in a clinical or clinical-adjacent leadership role. The key to the effectiveness of this role is ensuring that the person charged with leading the program has the desire, knowledge, and drive to lead the program using a collaborative, organization-wide approach.

3. **Establish or evaluate your violence prevention and de-escalation training program:** You probably already have some form of a de-escalation program in place within your organization. If you don't, now is the time to establish one and roll it out across the organization. A solid training program is key to empowering staff to keep themselves safe no matter where they work. When choosing a de-escalation program or evaluating your current one, here are some key considerations:

   a. Ensure that the program is through a recognized training provider and that it utilizes sound principles for both de-escalation and any physical techniques. Programs developed in-house that are "based on other programs" are not a good option from a variety of standpoints, especially regarding liability.

   b. The definition of workplace violence, types of workplace violence, national statistics, risk factors, situational awareness, and reporting procedures should be included in the course or through a supplemental course.

c. The program should be tailored or directly relevant to the healthcare environment whenever possible and not simply a generic course.

d. The program should utilize a tiered approach so that it can be rolled out to staff across the organization based on their risk level. For example, a cafeteria employee needs a basic-level online introductory course covering basic de-escalation skills, whereas a direct patient care provider in the emergency department needs a full course that includes in-person patient restraint techniques and self-defense options.

e. Training via online courses should be an option so that the training is readily accessible. However, physical skills training should always be conducted in person by a qualified trainer.

f. A train-the-trainer option should be available so that the organization can leverage its own instructors to teach the in-person portions of the course.

4. **Create a Threat Assessment/Management Team:** Threat assessment and management is one of the most powerful and cost-effective tools you can leverage to prevent and mitigate not only patient violence but violence by employees, visitors, and others. When establishing a threat assessment team and process or evaluating the one you currently have in place, here are some of the basic elements you should consider:

a. The team should be multidisciplinary and include leadership from security, human resources, risk management, legal, clinical operations, and patient relations.

b. Initial and ongoing training for how to assess and manage threats is essential for the team, and it should be provided by a recognized organization that employs an empirically validated structured assessment tool. Examples of this training/tools include, but are not limited to, the Workplace Assessment of Violence Risk (WAVR-21) and the Cawood Assessment Grid for Organizational (Workplace) Violence.

c. There should be a clear, written workflow for the team that is used to evaluate and manage threats.

d. A forensic psychologist or psychiatrist with expertise in threat assessment and management should be available to the team for consultation on an as-needed basis.

5. **Establish a Patient Behavioral Emergency Response and Management Framework:** While the threat assessment team is useful for evaluating potentially violent situations, a clinically based threat response and management framework should also be established that is available to clinical teams on a 24/7 basis. This threat response framework is not dependent on specific individuals like the threat assessment team; rather, it is made up of ad-hoc members based on their role/position who are normally available to respond at all times, such as the nursing administrator, security supervisor, psychiatrist on-call, the patient's nurse and the patient's current physician. Two examples of such frameworks are described below:

a. SAFE Response: Created by Brigham and Women's Hospital, the SAFE Response model has been proven to be an effective intervention strategy for escalating, potentially violent patients. SAFE stands for Spot a threat, Assess the risk, Formulate a safe plan, and Evaluate the outcome. The program includes mandatory training for all clinical staff on the SAFE model, standardized interventions, and a timely 24/7 team deployment availability through the hospital operator. A study evaluating the effectiveness of the program published in 2019 found that, after the program was implemented, "Nursing staff injury rates decreased an average of 40%" (Lakatos et al., 2019, p. 287).

b. Behavioral Emergency Response Team (BERT): While BERT teams are starting to gain support within hospital organizations across the United States, this effective approach with myriad benefits is not a widely adopted intervention strategy. An AMA Journal article examining the prevalence and use of BERT teams found that "The standardized emergency code suggestions of 21 state hospital associations fail to endorse a protocol for general behavioral emergencies that is distinct from security-only protocols" (Parker et al., 2020, p. 958). However, the benefits of the limited research available on these teams are clear. In fact, in one BERT implementation at the University of Maryland Medical Center, the results of the team's interventions were nothing short of outstanding. A study of the team's effectiveness across two years indicated that the team responded to 209 calls with no injuries reported and an average intervention time of thirty minutes (Noll & Doyle, 2017). In another study, a BERT team was launched for a three-month pilot on a medical-surgical unit where the team responded to 17 behavioral emergencies. The positive impacts of the team were evident in the results: "The number of assaults decreased from 10 (pre) to 1 (post); security intervention decreased from 14 to 1; and restraint use decreased from 8 to 1" (Zicko et al., 2017, p. 377). While more research into the effectiveness of these teams is needed, the initial results are promising. Further, with a flexible implementation model that places security in a supporting role rather than a primary role, clinicians are empowered to handle behavioral emergencies, and security resources are reserved for only times when they are truly needed.

6. **Investigate Incidents and Support Victims:** Every incident of patient violence should be investigated to determine the root cause (if known) and/or events preceding the incident, who was impacted by the violence, and whether follow-up action is required. The investigation may be cursory in nature or may be in-depth, depending on the circumstances and severity of the incident. While the security team may lead such investigations, it is important to collaborate with other stakeholders, such as human resources, risk management, and clinical leadership. Victims should be regularly updated on the status of the investigation to reassure them that the incident is being taken seriously. Consistent and transparent investigations into incidents of patient violence can also help encourage staff to report incidents more frequently, as the word will get out that reporting leads to follow-up and action.

   Further, victims of patient violence require the support of varying degrees depending on the type of violence, whether there was a physical and/or psychological injury, and the level of actual and/or perceived future risk experienced by the victim. Support may include a referral to the Employee Assistance Program, assistance with filing criminal charges and/or obtaining a protective order, a follow-up by the victim's manager and/or human resources, a personalized safety plan, and more.

7. **Mitigate Forensic Patient Risk:** Forensic patients, or patient prisoners, represent a threat to any healthcare organization since a hospital or other healthcare settings often represents a weak link in the chain of custody. Patient prisoners attempting to

escape custody have injured, raped, kidnapped, and murdered hospital and healthcare staff. These escape attempts, which are sometimes successful, are not rare events. A 2011 study funded by the International Healthcare Security and Safety Foundation found that, in a one-year span, there was a reported 99 forensic prisoner escapes in hospitals across the US (Mikow & Smith, 2011, p. 38).

It's critical to ensure that you not only have a solid policy and procedure regarding forensic patients but that you also maintain regular communications with local and state law enforcement, courts, and corrections leadership. Your policies and procedures would ring hollow with police and corrections officers with patient prisoners at your organization if the officers weren't informed of them by their own leadership. Further, security staff must serve as active liaisons with both personnel charged with maintaining the security of patient prisoners and with clinical staff caring for these patients.

8. **Get a Seat at the New Construction/Renovation Planning Table:** Leveraging the built environment to foster PVPM is a critical opportunity that is often missed by organizations due to a lack of awareness, good planning, and leaving security leadership out of the planning process. It is critical that security leadership is always plugged into the planning process, with a regular seat at the table, starting at the conceptual planning stage. The International Association of Healthcare Security and Safety (IAHSS) offers excellent resources for guidance in building security into the healthcare environment, including their publication, *Security Design Guidelines for Healthcare Facilities*.

9. **Create a Data Visualization Dashboard:** In order to keep tabs on your program's performance and effectiveness, it's important to continue to gather and analyze data relevant to patient violence and your prevention and mitigation strategies. One of the best ways to do this is by using a dashboard to help you visualize the data in a way that is easy to understand and digest. Using a dashboard also allows you to share the data and analyses with leaders and other key stakeholders who need to stay informed. Programs such as Microsoft Power BI and Tableau are commonly used to create dashboards, but there is a multitude of tools available online with varying

degrees of development difficulty. Chances are that there is someone within your organization with the skills and knowledge to build your custom dashboard. The dashboard should be updated monthly with new data and shared with appropriate persons within your organization.

Section 6. PVPM Program Step 4: Maintain

1. **Repeat the PVPM Program Steps:** The steps you followed in order to put your PVPM program into motion—Assess, Establish the Foundation, and Build—should be repeated on an annual basis to evaluate the effectiveness of your program. This doesn't mean that you need to start the process over from scratch, but rather review what you have built to ensure that it is effective in the face of any new information, data, organizational changes/challenges, or emerging threats. Here are some examples of how you might evaluate your program:

   a. Assess: Use the data you are collecting and analyzing to measure whether the program you have established is effective in achieving desired outcomes related to PVPM. Examples include a reduction in staff and patient injuries, a reduction in the use of restraints, and an increased use of behavioral emergency response and management interventions.

   b. Establish the Foundation: Is your program's foundation still solid? Your foundation may need to be firmed up if any of the following are true:

      i. There's been turnover in the C-Suite, and the new or interim leadership is not informed about/engaged in the PVPM program.

      ii. Your C-Suite champion has left the organization, is too busy to help, or has otherwise disengaged from the PVPM program.

      iii. Policies and procedures need to be updated.

      iv. Your workplace violence committee has stagnated.

      v. You have failed to consistently engage your communications team.

These are all just examples, of course. Other issues can impact the effectiveness of the PVPM program's foundation as well, so you should closely examine your foundation for signs of compromise and take steps to mitigate any issues you find.

c. Build: Take a look at what you have built so far on your foundation. What has been implemented to mitigate the risks you previously identified? Do you need to shift priorities based on emerging risks, lack of financial resources, or other issues? Have any efforts to build the PVPM stalled? Momentum is the key to any successful outcomes with the PVPM program, so any signs of a slowdown, dwindling interest, lack of engagement, or other issues detrimental to your program should be addressed.

2. **Conduct Ongoing Unit-Level Risk Assessments:** Your initial patient violence risk assessment shouldn't be the only time that you examine the physical and operational risks related to patient violence within your organization. Regular, ongoing inpatient and outpatient unit violence risk assessments are key to understanding PVPM challenges and opportunities within each unit. They also allow your team to gain a greater understanding of the operations within each unit while building relationships with the people who work in them. Don't limit your assessments to the day shift, either. Check out 24/7 units on the evening and night shifts as well since the nature of the operations and the related challenges can vary from shift to shift.

Ideally, these assessments should be conducted by a multidisciplinary group-preferably from the workplace violence committee, using an assessment tool the committee created for a consistent approach and information/data collection strategy. The bonus here is that your committee members will gain a new perspective on the unit, gain new skills, and make new connections with the people who work on the unit. The committee members conducting the assessment should also make recommendations for improvements before submitting it to the full committee for follow-up. Recommendations should be prioritized like the initial assessment you conducted at the start of the PVPM program, and follow-up action on these recommendations is essential.

3. **Leverage Micro-Training:** Micro-training is essentially a mini-drill that can be conducted by a member of the security team or clinical team with one or more staff

members within an inpatient or outpatient setting. This type of training is helpful for keeping staff skills around patient violence prevention and mitigation fresh. After all, according to the Ebbinghaus forgetting curve and subsequent research into this phenomenon, "learners will forget on average 90% of material within 1 month" (Woolliscroft, 2020, p. 250). However, this research has also revealed that "…revisiting material at regular intervals, whether through presentations, electronic communication, or testing, enhances retention" (Woolliscroft, 2020, p. 257). In order to ensure that staff de-escalation skills and related patient violence prevention and mitigation skills stay front-of-mind, regular, bite-sized refresher opportunities are essential.

Micro-training typically consists of a scenario presented to the participant, followed by questions for the participant to answer. After the participant answers the questions, this provides an opportunity to educate the participant on the correct responses or additional options for handling the situation. Gathering a small group of participants can further enhance the learning experience as they can bounce ideas off of one another. An example of micro-training is included in the appendix.

Section 7. PVPM Program Next Steps

Now that you have read the entire PVPM program outline return to the "assess" step and start the process of building your own program within your organization. Take the process in small chunks, as it's easy to get overwhelmed with this type of work. Don't forget to work with a multidisciplinary team and get the right people to support you and the team's efforts. You can do this!

Conclusion

I sincerely hope that this manual provides you with the information, guidance, and motivation you need to move forward with building an effective, sustainable patient violence prevention and mitigation program. Whether you have a program in place already or you are starting from scratch, your work on this issue is so vitally important.

You play such an important role in ensuring that hospital staff and others are safe from violence. When the threat of violence is no longer something that staff must constantly fear, they can focus on what matters most, which is patient care. In essence, the program you are working to build will have the greatest impact on those your organization serves and the quality of care they receive. What could be a greater payoff?

So, move forward with a bias for action with a basis in data. Ask for help to build your program starting from the top—don't do it alone. Persevere in the face of the mounting complexity, evolution, and persistence of violence. Stay the course and "build the house" with a solid foundation that will endure for many years to come. Don't get distracted by urges within yourself or from others to waste time or energy on quick fixes. Your role in leading the charge is critical.

Thank you again for everything you are doing—small and large—to make your organization safer. I am truly grateful for your work, and so are those whom you serve.

APPENDIX

Glossary

Patient Violence

Violence in any form committed by a person who is receiving care is registered to receive care and/or has previously received care from a healthcare organization.

Patient Violence Prevention and Mitigation (PVPM) Program

Coordinated efforts undertaken by a healthcare organization in order to prevent patient violence from occurring and/or to mitigate the impacts of patient violence. These efforts can take many forms- from policy to training and environmental planning.

Workplace Violence

According to the ANSI/ASIS International Workplace Violence and Active Assailant-Prevention, Intervention, and Response standard, workplace violence is defined as "A spectrum of behaviors, including overt acts of violence, threats, and other conduct that generates a reasonable concern for safety from violence, where a nexus exists between the behavior and the physical safety of employees from any internal or external relationship" (ANSI/ASIS International, 2020, p. 8).

Workplace Violence Mitigation

Measures taken by an organization to reduce the impact of violence on staff, patients, visitors, and others. These measures may include providing a rapid response by a security team or Behavioral Emergency Response Team (BERT), offering counseling services after an incident, or developing a safety plan for a victim of threats.

Workplace Violence Prevention

Any efforts by an organization to stop violence before it happens by employing means such as staff training, patient screening, environmental security and safety elements, and more.

Micro-Training Example

Aggressive Patient Scenario

Instructions: Approach staff who do not appear to be busy with patient care or other duties. Ask if they have 2–3 minutes to spare to run through a quick scenario-based training with you. Explain the scenario and then ask them what they would do if they were to encounter the situation in their area right now. Then, educate them on the options for response to the situation as outlined within this document.

After running through the training, be sure to record the names of the participants, job titles, practice locations, and whether they found the training to be helpful. If possible, hold this training with small (2–4 people) groups of staff.

Scenario: Imagine that right this minute, a patient who has been somewhat agitated while in the waiting room leaps out of his chair and aggressively approaches the reception desk. He starts screaming and demanding that someone get his doctor right away. He says he doesn't have any more time to wait, and he needs his medications. Other patients and staff appear visibly concerned by his outburst. Walk through the steps of how you would respond to this situation.

Options for Response: Here are some options for responding to this type of situation. Your response will ultimately be dictated by the situation at the moment.

1. Create distance between yourself and the patient- at least 4+ feet.

2. Leave the reception desk and go to a safer location within the practice if needed.

3. Summon a co-worker to help you.

4. If it is safe to do so, attempt to engage the patient verbally at a safe distance to de-escalate him.

5. Call security or ask a co-worker to call security if you can't do so safely. Activate the duress alarm if you have one.

References

Alzheimer's Association. *Aggression and Anger*. Available from: https://www.alz.org/help-support/caregiving/stages-behaviors/agression-anger#:~:text=It%20is%20not%20uncommon%20for,express%20it%20through%20physical%20aggression.

American Psychological Association. (n.d.). *Socioeconomic status*. American Psychological Association. Retrieved September 13, 2022, from https://www.apa.org/topics/socioeconomic-status

ANSI/ASIS International. *Workplace Violence and Active Assailant- Prevention, Intervention, and Response Standard*. 2020 May.

Anthony A. Braga; William H. Sousa; James R. Coldren, Jr.; and Denise Rodriguez, The Effects of Body-Worn Cameras on Police Activity and Police-Citizen Encounters: A Randomized Controlled Trial, 108 *Journal of Criminal Law & Criminology* 511 (2018). https://scholarlycommons.law.northwestern.edu/jclc/vol108/iss3/3

Arnetz JE, Hamblin L, Essenmacher L, Upfal MJ, Ager J, Luborsky M. Understanding patient-to-worker violence in hospitals: a qualitative analysis of documented incident reports. *Journal of Advanced Nursing*. 2015 Feb;71(2):338-48. doi: 10.1111/jan.12494. Epub 2014 Aug 4. PMID: 25091833; PMCID: PMC5006065.

Averill, R. F., Mills, R. E. (2021, November). *Socioeconomic status and health care delivery system performance*. Retrieved September 13, 2022, from https://multimedia.3m.com/mws/media/2117913O/his-pm-cer-socioeconomic-status-health-care-delivery-system-performance-report-en-us.pdf

Barak Ariel et al., Wearing Body-Cameras Increases Assaults Against Officers and Do Not Reduce Police-Use of Force: Results from a Global Multisite Experiment, 13 *European Journal of Criminology* 744, 750 (2016).

Borofsky LA, Kellerman I, Baucom B, Oliver PH, Margolin G. Community Violence Exposure and Adolescents' School Engagement and Academic Achievement Over

Time. *Psychology of Violence*. 2013 Oct 1;3(4):381-395. doi: 10.1037/a0034121. PMID: 24163782; PMCID: PMC3806333.

Brusie, C. (n.d.). *Nurse dies after being attacked by mental health patient - manslaughter charges*. Nurse.org. Retrieved October 16, 2022, from https://nurse.org/articles/nurse-attacked-by-patient-dies-manslaughter/

C. Noll, K. Doyle. *Behavioral emergency response team: implementing a performance improvement strategy to address workplace violence* [Internet]. University of Maryland Medical Center. Available from: https://ancc.confex.com/ancc/ANCCMagnet2015/webprogram/Handout/Paper15064/p1008.pdf [cited 2022 Sep 18]

FBI. (2019, September 13). *Murder*. FBI. Retrieved September 28, 2022, from https://ucr.fbi.gov/crime-in-the-u.s/2019/crime-in-the-u.s.-2019/topic-pages/murder

FBI. (2019, September 13). *Rape*. FBI. Retrieved September 28, 2022, from https://ucr.fbi.gov/crime-in-the-u.s/2019/crime-in-the-u.s.-2019/topic-pages/rape#:~:text=The%20revised%20UCR%20definition%20of,the%20consent%20of%20the%20victim.

Garcia-Arocena, D. *The genetics of violent behavior*. 2015. Available from: https://www.jax.org/news-and-insights/jax-blog/2015/december/the-genetics-of-violent-behavior

Hall, R. C. W., Hall, R. C. W., Chapman, M. J. (2009, January). *Nursing Home Violence: Occurrence, Risks, and Interventions*. Hmpgloballearningnetwork.com. Retrieved September 11, 2022, https://www.hmpgloballearningnetwork.com/site/altc/content/nursing-home-violence-occurrence-risks-and-interventions#:~:text=Nursing%20assistants%20working%20in%20long,the%20nursing%20home%20(NH).

Harvard University Center on the Developing Child. *Executive Function and Self Regulation*. Available from: https://developingchild.harvard.edu/science/key-concepts/executive-function/

NAMI. *Here are Nami's three steps for being StigmaFree*. (n.d.). Retrieved September 11, 2022, from https://www.nami.org/Get-Involved/Pledge-to-Be-StigmaFree

Hersh K, Borum R. Command hallucinations, compliance, and risk assessment. *Journal of the American Academy of Psychiatry and the Law.* 1998;26(3):353-9. PMID: 9785279.

Im DS. Template to Perpetrate: An Update on Violence in Autism Spectrum Disorder. *Harvard Review of Psychiatry.* 2016 Jan-Feb;24(1):14-35. doi: 10.1097/ HRP.0000000000000087. PMID: 26735321; PMCID: PMC4710161.

James O. Woolliscroft, Chapter 19 - Considerations when designing educational experiences, Editor(s): James O. Woolliscroft, *Implementing Biomedical Innovations into Health, Education, and Practice.* Academic Press, 2020, Pages 249-260.

Knaak S, Mantler E, Szeto A. Mental illness-related stigma in healthcare: Barriers to access and care and evidence-based solutions. *Healthcare Management Forum.* 2017 Mar;30(2):111-116. doi: 10.1177/0840470416679413. Epub 2017 Feb 16. PMID: 28929889; PMCID: PMC5347358.

Krakowski, M. Violence and Serotonin: Influence of Impulse Control, Affect Regulation, and Social Functioning. *Journal of Neuropsychiatry and Clinical Neurosciences.* 1 Aug 2003. Available from: https://neuro.psychiatryonline.org/doi/10.1176/ jnp.15.3.294#:~:text=Serotonin%20is%20seen%20as%20playing,both%20 violence%20and%20impulse%20control.

Lakatos BE, Mitchell MT, Askari R, Etheredge ML, Hopcia K, DeLisle L, Smith C, Fagan M, Mulloy D, Lewis-O'Connor A, Higgins M, Shellman A. An Interdisciplinary Clinical Approach for Workplace Violence Prevention and Injury Reduction in the General Hospital Setting: S.A.F.E. Response. *Journal of the American Psychiatric Nurses Association.* 2019 Jul/Aug;25(4):280-288. doi: 10.1177/1078390318788944. Epub 2018 Jul 16. PMID: 30009653.

Mikow-Porto VA, Smith TA. The IHSSF 2011 Prisoner Escape Study. *Journal of Healthcare Protection Management.* 2011;27(2):38-58. PMID: 21916283.

Moore TJ, Glenmullen J, Furberg CD. Prescription drugs associated with reports of violence towards others. *PLoS One.* 2010 Dec 15;5(12):e15337. doi: 10.1371/ journal.pone.0015337. PMID: 21179515; PMCID: PMC3002271.

Norman, S., Elbogen, E. B., Schnurr, P. P. (2014, April 4). Va.gov: *Veterans Affairs. Research Findings on PTSD and Violence.* Retrieved September 10, 2022, from https://www.ptsd.va.gov/professional/treat/cooccurring/research_violence.asp#:~:text=Although%20PTSD%20is%20associated%20with,PTSD%20and%20violence%20is%20decreased.

Parker, C. B., Calhoun, A., Wong, A. H., Davidson, L., Dike, C. (2020, November 1). A call for behavioral emergency response teams in inpatient hospital settings. *Journal of Ethics | American Medical Association.* Retrieved September 18, 2022, from https://journalofethics.ama-assn.org/article/call-behavioral-emergency-response-teams-inpatient-hospital-settings/2020-11

Perkins, C., Beecher, D., Aberg, D.C. et al. Personal security alarms for the prevention of assaults against healthcare staff. *Crime Science* 6, 11 (2017). https://doi.org/10.1186/s40163-017-0073-1

Pitts E, Schaller DJ. Violent Patients. [Updated 2022 Mar 9]. In: *StatPearls* [Internet]. Treasure Island (FL): StatPearls Publishing; 2022 Jan-. Available from: https://www.ncbi.nlm.nih.gov/books/NBK537281/

Piza, E., Welsh, B., Farrington, D. and Thomas, A. (2019). CCTV Surveillance for Crime Prevention: A 40-Year Systematic Review with Meta-Analysis. *Criminology & Public Policy*, 18(1): 135-159.

Roy, E. (2013). Cognitive Impairment. In: Gellman, M.D., Turner, J.R. (eds) *Encyclopedia of Behavioral Medicine.* Springer, New York, NY. https://doi.org/10.1007/978-1-4419-1005-9_1118

Sarkar J. Borderline personality disorder and violence. *Australasian Psychiatry.* 2019;27(6):578-580. doi:10.1177/1039856219878644

Scott CL and Resnick PJ: Clinical assessment of aggression and violence. *Principles and Practice of Forensic Psychiatry, Third Edition* (Editors: Rosner R and Scott CL); CRC Press, Taylor & Francis Group, New York, 2017, pp 623-632.

Soreff SM, Gupta V, Wadhwa R, et al. Aggression. [Updated 2022 May 3]. In: *StatPearls* [Internet]. Treasure Island (FL): StatPearls Publishing; 2022 Jan-. Available from: https://www.ncbi.nlm.nih.gov/books/NBK448073/

Sussex Publishers. (n.d.). *Intermittent explosive disorder*. Psychology Today. Retrieved September 11, 2022, from https://www.psychologytoday.com/us/conditions/intermittent-explosive-disorder

Victim Connect Resource Center. *Stalking*. (2021, March 22). Retrieved September 28, 2022, from https://victimconnect.org/learn/types-of-crime/stalking/

The Joint Commission. (2021, June 18). R3 Report Issue 30: *Violence Prevention Standards*. Retrieved September 20, 2022, from https://www.jointcommission.org/-/media/tjc/documents/standards/r3-reports/wpvp-r3-30_revised_06302021.pdf

Va.gov: Veterans Affairs. *How Common is PTSD in Children and Teens?* (2018, September 18). Retrieved September 10, 2022, from https://www.ptsd.va.gov/understand/common/common_children_teens.asp#:~:text=Learn%20how%20many%20children%20and%20teenagers%20have%20PTSD.&text=Studies%20show%20that%20about%2015,certain%20types%20of%20trauma%20survivors.

Va.gov: Veterans Affairs. *How Common is PTSD in Adults?* (2018, September 13). Retrieved September 10, 2022, from https://www.ptsd.va.gov/understand/common/common_adults.asp#:~:text=Facts%20About%20How%20Common%20PTSD,PTSD%20during%20a%20given%20year.

Varshney M, Mahapatra A, Krishnan V, et al. Violence and mental illness: what is the true story? *Journal of Epidemiology and Community Health* 2016;70:223-225.

Zahoor I, Shafi A, Haq E. Pharmacological Treatment of Parkinson's Disease. In: Stoker TB, Greenland JC, editors. *Parkinson's Disease: Pathogenesis and Clinical Aspects* [Internet]. Brisbane (AU): Codon Publications; 2018 Dec 21. Chapter 7. Available from: https://www.ncbi.nlm.nih.gov/books/NBK536726/ doi: 10.15586/codonpublications.parkinsonsdisease.2018.ch7

Zicko CJM, Schroeder LRA, Byers CWS, Taylor LAM, Spence CDL. Behavioral Emergency Response Team: Implementation Improves Patient Safety, Staff Safety, and Staff Collaboration. *Worldviews on Evidence Based Nursing*. 2017 Oct;14(5):377-384. doi: 10.1111/wvn.12225. Epub 2017 Apr 3. PMID: 28372033.

ABOUT THE AUTHOR

David Corbin, Owner and Principal Consultant at the consulting firm Dynamic Security Strategies, LLC, has honed his specialization in private security over more than two decades. Using creativity and innovation, he has built highly effective security operations in several challenging environments from the ground up. Most recently, as the first Director of Campus Security Operations at Broad Institute of MIT and Harvard, he expanded the sophistication of security operations and workplace violence prevention efforts while supporting the organization's critical role as a regional COVID-19 test processing center. David also previously served as the Director of Police, Security and Parking at Brigham and Women's Hospital/Brigham Health, where he initiated a complete transformation of the 125-person Police & Security department from a contract security team to a proprietary team. As an Adjunct Professor at the Northeastern University School of Criminology and Criminal Justice, David developed and taught security management courses.

David is a member of the ASIS International Diversity, Equity and Inclusion Task Force and has been published in Campus Safety Magazine and the IAHSS Journal of Healthcare Protection Management. Under his leadership, the Police & Security Department at Faulkner Hospital won the prestigious Lindberg Bell Award in 2011 for establishing and maintaining an outstanding security program. He is also the 2016 recipient of the IAHSS Philip A. Gaffney Faculty Chair Award for his writings and works toward the furtherance of professionalism in the healthcare security field.

David holds credentials as a Certified Protection Professional (CPP), Certified Healthcare Protection Administrator (CHPA), and Certified Crime Prevention Through Environmental Design (CPTED) Specialist. He is a graduate of both the Gavin de Becker & Associates Advanced Threat Assessment and Management Academy and the Wharton/ASIS Security Executive Program. David holds a master's degree in Criminal Justice from Northeastern University in Boston, MA and a bachelor's degree in Criminal Justice from Roger Williams University in Bristol, RI.

He consults nationally on healthcare, K-12, higher education, government, and corporate security.

About Dynamic Security Strategies, LLC

Dynamic Security Strategies, LLC is an independent security consulting firm. We don't sell security equipment, products, or security labor services and are not affiliated with any vendor. Our firm comprises security practitioners with over 50 years of combined experience who have built and managed security operations for some of the most prestigious healthcare organizations in the United States. We are up-to-date on the latest risks and threats facing many organizations and are experienced in applying solutions to mitigate them. We have applied this knowledge to consulting engagements ranging from risk assessments at large multi-hospital systems, K-12 schools, municipal facilities, and private organizations, and building security into a $52M hospital campus expansion project.

Further, we have extensive experience in developing workplace violence prevention and mitigation programs, from policy writing to training and threat assessment. As practitioners who have fielded these programs, we know what strategies work and which ones don't work in today's environment. As consultants, we have assessed workplace violence risk at various organizations and developed prevention solutions customized for each organization.

Lastly, we are experienced educators and trainers who have served as long-term Adjunct Faculty at Northeastern University's School of Criminology and Criminal Justice. We also have a great deal of experience teaching security-related training programs and developing in-house training on topics such as workplace violence prevention and active shooter response.

In summary, we are uniquely qualified as consultants, practitioners, and educators to assess and mitigate your organization's risk and to develop solid training programs for your staff.